chapter one

Where do we begin well in a nutshell in 2002 a the age of 18 I decided I wanted to be a nurse there was no space in the mental health degree but there was on the learning disability one and i got my place.

I trained for 3 years and worked with many people with Autism through that training. I as a qualified nurse worked with Autistic individuals daily , understood various behaviours co-existing physical and mental health conditions and felt I understood Autism .

By 2011 I was about to have my second child and had worked at my then job for 6 years. I worked in an Autism unit prided myself on my job and was fascinated by the variety of patients I got to work with.

Now let me telL you a secret as an experienced nurse working in a specialist Autism unit the reality is I knew nothing about Autism until It decided to flip my world upside down.

My second child Olly joe was born on June 9th 2011 after a traumatic birth. I tell you this because so many people with Autism were born following a traumatic birth now I am no doctor but feel qualified enough to suggest that this may be a link to the condition.

Olly joe was in special care for a few days and when we took him home i am pretty sure all he did was get sick and cry. This again may seem useless information but it is known that children with Autism have more sleep problems than other children in a nutshell our brain release melatonin to help us sleep….

Autistic people often don't produce any or enough melatonin and sleep disturbance can be caused. Was Olly-Joe simply a sick baby as my mother would say or was it an early indicator of Autism… lots of research argues that children with Autism often also have gastro-intestinal problems. I Was blessed no sleep and constantly covered in sick. I was even more blessed with some of the useless advice people felt it was ok to dish out one family member suggested I get hold of some phennygen to 'make him sleep hmmmmm I was mortified and for the do gooders waiting to pounce no I never followed that advice for your information I am still bloody shattered and need a weeks sleep .

Maybe he is hungry, maybe he is cold.. I heard it all I am not stupid I said to Lee one day do people think I bloody well enjoy being a zombie and getting no sleep I vented.

As my maternity leave ticked away so did my energy and life became a blur of trying to get sleep me and lee regularly took turns on the sofa to get a sleep. Dempsie my oldest tearfully asked me one day if her brother could go back to the hospital because she needed some sleep. My heart broke for her she was just 3 when she said this. GP's gave me all sorts of explanations, he had acid reflux he had a milk allergy, he just did not need sleep.

I was so so tired I thought I was losing my mind. I forgot things off shopping lists missed appointments was never on time for anything and hardly saw my friends.

pressure on relationships is difficult with any baby let alone an insomniac vomiting machine.

I kicked lee out in a stressed tired rage one day I decided he was useless (he's not he is actually a bloody brilliant Dad even if I think he is a dick sometimes) and I was too tired to hear him out off he went to his Mother's. As usual I was labelled the bad one by others so called friends even messaged him to see if he was ok. Kelly the apparent psychopath who was no good for him was simply at breaking point you nosey cows safe to say I've lost a lot of useless friends along the way.

This was more than a newborn baby this was 2 hours maximum sleep a day constant bouts of your baby getting unwell all the time and basically feeling like it would never end. This was feeling like a bad mother on a daily basis because all your baby did was cry.

Maternity leave over and it became time to get back to work. I was back a week and a male staff member was rude to me over something trivial and made me cry. He apologised but after 9 months of no sleep I wasn't ready to listen I had an almighty strop that under normal circumstances would be totally disproportionate even for a stroppy cow like me . I got moved to another ward at the hospital that was shorter shifts and less busy. I have toughened up if I was spoken to like that these days the response would be totally different, I would totally utilise the robust policies of the organisation I work for nobody goes to work to be spoken to like they are dirt even if in hindsight I over reacted.

I settled but Olly joe hated nursery he just couldn't settle wouldn't play with other babies and screamed if staff looked at him. I made a decision 3 months later to just juggle shifts and childcare. Night shifts were my preference I figured I was always awake anyway, the money was good and it helped with childcare Lee really realised why I was like a deranged cow when he started having to deal with not sleeping when I was doing nights.

2 nights and one morning a week I worked it killed me but the bill needed paying.
People asked me how I did it , I remember saying to a colleague once well I Cant send him back can I. They looked horrified but the reality is no matter how difficult things are your kids are your kids.

18 months old Olly had a check up .. they were concerned about his development and he was referred to a centre. I had the usual oh he is fine, oh he is a boy, oh he just don't like sleep from family that meant well but did not have to function on no sleep. This centre offered an appointment but it was in 12 months time I plodded on as you do.

We moved house in the process of getting ready to finally get married so that appointment never happened.

2 years and 3 months we got married and when I tell you my son never coped he never coped. I never said my vows in peace he was literally on my hip. I look back at some of our photo's and he just looks lost.

My Mother couldn't get him dressed at the time I was fuming at her the reality is Olly hates fitted clothes so a mini wedding suit and waistcoat was never going to be favourable with him. I felt helpless as He cried most of the day in fact one of the most poignant photos of my day was of me collapsed in a heap shattered at 9pm took on a friends phone . 230 guests, noise a disco and his mum in a dress and looking human for once was merely a shock to his system. This is one of the hardest parts of being an Autism parent…joyous occasions to other people become an absolute battlefield for you and your family we nowadays select carefully which parties we go to . The day after a party or wedding is always hard for Olly I believe it simply takes him longer to process all the noise and hustle and bustle than other people. Olly has been known to literally cry all day after a party hence why we are so selective. I refuse to distress my child for a whole 24 hours for a 3 hour party. iI do however attend a few with him because the reality is the world is not made for autism it is not understanding . Ear defenders a weighted blanket a full change of clothes. A picture of where we are going shown days before are all part and parcel of what we do to understand our little boy. I never knew all this when we got married to this day it hurts me how stressed he was that day.

Those of you with children on the spectrum sod what everyone else thinks if your special occasions involve your child… it's simple it has to be accommodating .. they are already trying to make sense of their world . Parties now we are selective with and have to plan with military precision. I have some amazing friends that offer a quiet space when they're children have parties my family have weddings christenings funerals at a local club regularly. Everyone knows we always sit at the same table it is just easier for Olly a table furthest away from the noise of the dj playing his cheesy pop.

Nursery

So after a long break we attempted another nursery when I tell you my son does not like small people I am not joking i mean he literally attacked kids and teachers galore yet was happy at home sat playing with the same toy for hours. Olly's speech was a lot slower to develop even at 2 and a half he wasn't really speaking.

I thought it would get better it seemed to practically overnight.... until a doctor spoke to me about echolalia ... my sons speech was behind but he was able to mimic conversations he had heard. He was parroting what he had heard. I am pleased to say he hasn't called his Dad a dick or a a moron yet so my language is clearly improving.

Nursery got repainted one day Olly had to be collected he was hysterical and kept pointing at the walls they thought he was poorly the reality was he was raging that the environment had changed still Autism was not at the forefront of my mind. Even if it was people would just tell me he was fine he would grow out if it

Not a week went by without an incident Olly was eventually placed in a room with just one other child and he became happier an outbursts were less frequent. Toilet training was a no go we tried believe me .. he just could not get the timing right i have on so many occasions had to comfort my child who so desperately wants to get to the toilet but doesn't quite make it there has been a vicious cycle of constipation .. followed by rectal digging all the stuff people don't actually realise comes as part and parcel of some children with autism.

Autism is an arsehole at times for this simple reason you can be going weeks with your child getting on ok with everything no incontinence no issues at school then bang a week of meltdowns incidents anxiety and incontinence reminds you why your child got a diagnosis. I have joked when Olly has had a really bad day the if Autism was a person I would kick it in the crotch. Not all children are incontinent not all children have anxiety as well this is just our example.

Assessment

At the time we started getting appointments for assessment a well known British soap had a storyline where after one a appointment a chid was diagnosed as having ADHD and prescribed medication . I am telling you now even private assessments do not work like that.

9 appointments in all we had from school observations to home visits to us being sat in a centre with other parents being observed. I was convinced the whole time I was a bad Mother my confidence was so low. I was able to for the first time see what happens in an Autism assessment …despite my job i had always managed people who already had an Autism diagnosis so this was not something I had prior knowledge of.

I watched as my little boy literally ran away from the other children in the assessment he just did not want to play he was happiest sat alone. When the clinicians attempted to play with him he denied to tell them he had a bad belly and needed a doctor.

I was told to complete sleep diaries and my children evening routine scrutinised I felt like my child having a poor sleep pattern made me a criminal of some sort.

The team were struck by Olly's inability to sit still for long and fascinated by his so called photographic memory.

Even the play at assessments is very staged it is how they complete them totally not like the movies and soaps and nothing like some of the rubbish i have read online.

Diagnosis

After all the appointments were completed we were called back. A report of every second of those assessments was given to us I wept as I read through all the difficulties. This single moment made me vow to include positives on any nursing report I then had to write for child or a young person. I knew he struggled I knew we were there for a reason but I never knew how much he struggled.

A lovely Doctor then came to give her opinion on our son

Then came the words we have reached a decision and Olly meets the criteria for Autistic Spectrum disorder. I wept I had never been so angry, angry at each and every person who had thought i was mad the so called friends who had thought I was bat shit crazy wen actually I was exhausted. The family who had no contact with us , the colleagues who thought I did not know they spent their damn night shifts debating whether I was crazy or if my son was difficult.

Lee hugged me and I calmly told him I had thought I was going mad and was relieved we had some answers as to why things at times are so difficult for our lad. Now I would love to write how good the post diagnostic support was but it wasn't a 5 week introduction to Autism course was offered that only accommodated non-working parents, A disability benefits leaflet and some wonderful sleep diaries and we were waved up the path.

Dempsie-Lee (Dem)

Dempsie lee was 6 when Olly got diagnosed we told her that her brothers brain works differently to other little boys brains. Dem matter factly asked me . Does Daddy have Autism then your always telling him to get things into his brain. I roared with laughter.

Dem is 8 as I write this she can put a lot of adults to shame with her compassion towards other children with disabilities. Her best friend is a local little girl wheelchair bound with no verbal speech. Dem informs me that her little friend can talk with her eyes and will spend hours talking to her in fact she told me just the other day just because someone does not speak does not mean they cannot listen. I think my daughter is amazeballs .

My little superstar asked me if she could help with this book so here is her view on Autism in her own words.

my name is Dempsie-Lee Stone
my brother is Autistic he can't deal with plans being changed, sometimes he gets his words back to front so he says he is hot but he is cold. My brother only likes beige foods. My brother hits people sometimes I think it is hard for people with Autism because they think differently .

My 8 year old… just totally summed up Autism in a few sentences yet I meet so called professionals who think they've nailed Autism and don;t have her level of compassion  the difference is my daughter lives with someone with Autism and she wants to understand. When more people want to understand we will be in a better place.

Attitudes.

Here is a list of responses I got at Olly being diagnosed these responses are from family friends colleagues such as Doctor's nurses yes in 2016 we still have a long way to go with attitudes .

'he will grow out of it'
'Diagnosis is just the start of your journey'
'he doesn't have it bad'
'he does not look autistic'
'maybe they have got it wrong'
'maybe his injections caused it'
'will your daughter be tested because of it being contagious'
'Will he be ok at school'
'will he need medication'
'My network marketing overpriced tablets may help'

No I never slapped anybody because there is a difference between miseducation and malice.

Am I angry ? No

My energy whats left after no sleep…. is used wisely I would help anyone who approached me for advice around ASD no i am not a doctor no i am not an expert. However I am an expert by experience of how it feels what to do and where to go. Being nice really costs nothing.

literal thinking

Olly is very literal and we have had some laughter and tears here are some examples.

'Dad you smell desperate' this came after him hearing me tell my husband he was desperate for a shower.

'Dad does grandad live in the night garden'. my dad works abroad on boats a lot. A character from the night garden also lives in a boat.

'mom I won't get any christmas presents I am sad'... upon realising there is no visible chimney on our roof '

We saw a young black man riding a horse Olly now believes every black man he meets has a pet horse and gets quite irate when informed someone does not have a horse.

'Look at my mums belly there is a baby in there' my que to get back to fat club was given.

Olly can you put your pants on son. Followed by him putting them on over his dirty ones. Note taken to break things down into small exact steps.

food

Nuggets, chips, rice bananas only if they don't have a spot on.

ice cream vanilla only. Mash fish fingers chicken.

Believe me we have tried, we have offered new items regularly but unless it is beige he generally just won't have it.

My advice speak to your gp get some vitamins and pick your battles with food wisely .

My son would literally not eat if the wrong food was offered We just keep trying I liquidise a lot of veg into a sauce and freeze portions so of he ever asks for anything with gravy, sauce or baked beans which he will do literally once a month there is always some vegetables hidden in the food.

Olly likes his food to not touch i had a lot of dinners thrown up walls before being able to see that this was a problem.

There are 2 restaurants he will eat in one is an indian restaurant where everything he orders is beige, dry and offered on separate plates.

The second is a buffet place, he chooses what goes on his plate so that works well.

School dinner time is hell on earth most of his incidents have been around mealtime we reduced this by 70 percent by trying him on packed lunches. The reason being … he knows what is in them and it is less anxiety provoking for him.

I have had heated discussions with lee who gets stressed if the kids don't eat one morning he asked Olly 8 times to eat. if you asked me who is not diagnosed as Autistic 8 times I would be fuming consequently i blew at him and told him he was a nause and that Olly would eat when he was hungry. Olly still calls his dad a nause when asked to eat his dinner to this day.

I think to myself even now how boring it must be having nuggets every time you eat out. I then remind myself how hard we try to vary his diet and how common it actually is for children on the spectrum to have restricted diets. In fact ask any professional working in eating disorders how many children with undiagnosed Autism actually enter eating disorder services because of their extreme rigid diets.

I often think of hospital environments who only have limited menu ideas and cannot offer a restricted diet to their patients on the spectrum another example of how our society and resources need to think outside the box to offer individuals with Autistic Spectrum disorder as calm and routinely a stay as possible.

I can recall incidents in my professional life of those with Autism becoming so stressed around mealtimes they become violent I now understand this more and would love to roll out some form of education programme to help others to see through an Autistic persons eyes.

The hard part

Family will tell you that its because you spoil them, employers will be disgusted that you need another day off for another meeting. I count my blessings where employment is concerned as Olly was being diagnosed I had an amazing Doctor and nurse manager who worked my workload around his appointments. in fact I Left that job to progress, in reality I should have stayed where I was they understood Autism and emphaphised with me when I was getting phoned by nurseries , schools , childminders and babysitters about the latest incident. I am not going to say anything is easy because quite frankly Autism sucks at times.

In fact as I may have mentioned before there are days Autism requires a good kick in the balls for the anxiety it ignites in my little boy and in many other people on the spectrum.

the theres watching your child develop a skill then lose it. I have watched skills learned then disappear overnight .

The sensory element can pretty much suck too. Parties, loud noises bright lights, clothing , seatbelt have caused anxiety so high in my child that he has hit kicked punched and spat and been labelled a naughty boy. A family friend told me my son maybe needed more discipline I said maybe you need less ignorance.

Getting halfway to a destination to realise you've packed forgotten your child's ear defenders the M6 services don't stock these sort of items. Toothpaste , deodorant your fine.

Then theres the bowel issues that can time limit accessing certain places.

Believe me it is not all hard my pride for my children makes me smile inside I mean we live in a world where we expect everyone to fit into a generic box. I admire the fact Olly don't care about what people think yes he lacks self awareness yes he blurts out things he shouldn't but would I ever change him….no because Autism is simply an explanation not what defines him in fact I believe the world would be boring if we was all the robots the mainstream media and government wants us to be.

My son can direct you from Birmingham to somerset without hesitating , he can name the model of most cars that drive past. He is funny.

My daughter at the age of 8 wants to write an ebook on how it feels to be a sibling of someone society labels as different she will tell you everybody is the same on the inside .

advice

Fail to plan and plan to fail . We plan everything in advance . We try to stick to a reasonable routine even in school holidays.

Pick your battles undesirable behaviour is totally different to unmanageable behaviour sometimes we need to lower our expectations.

Forget what people think . No child comes with a manual no child is perfect even experienced professionals don't live with Autism life won't be perfect just do your best to enter their world.

Analyse. Most incidents your child has will have a reason its worth logging it down eventually you pick out triggers and change how you do things. My sons broke noses chipped teeth dented walls and doors, but perseverance means his incidents are now few and far between and we can dampen things down quite quickly. We are not perfect , we are working class parents that like a night off here and there to let our hair down or even ore importantly catch up on sleep.

obsessions - A lot of Autistic children will have obsessions, allow them some structured time to talk about them as actually shutting them down can make them more anxious. For example Olly loves cars and would talk to you all day about engines, colours brands models. We have a routine of walking our dogs where he can point out cars talk about them matter of factly without getting himself worked up. Sometimes we simply need to adapt.

School- Personally i found ofsted rating means nothing staffs ability to answer questions on their special needs provision examples and talking to other parents helps. Fight for everything your child needs you are their eyes and if even you can't always make sense of their behaviour why would someone not related to them. Give school as much information as possible.
My kids school isn't rated as fantastic but is always striving to do better schools that need to improve are sometimes trying harder to get things right then those ho have became complacent.  I am not an expert in schools but the feel of the school was the most important thing to me. one highly rated school couldn't answer my questions on their Autism provisions so it was a no.

listen to your gut- I ignored mine when my lad was  a baby and caused myself so much heartache when the reality was the early signs of Autism were there.

hospital

Another fine example of my sons antics one Saturday he decided he wanted to get inside the tv because thats what happens in Charlie and he chlorate factory he smashed a 32 inch tv over his head resulting in a trip to the local children's hospital.

Have you ever been to A and E with s chid whom hates bright lights, loud noises and strange places. Have you ever had your child completely trash a visitors lounge then vomit now a chid who has had a tv land on his head vomiting means an overnight stay in hospital. When I mean it was exhausting it really was I am pretty sure that they could not wait to discharge us. Poor kid screamed constantly cried begged for the automated lights to be off . The tuts the stares, the dirty looks off other parents were lovely I must admit.

I started a petition that night about waiting areas in A and E needing to be more disabled friendly. I got loads of abuse because I sated in the petition children wth special needs and was accused of forgetting adults. Not one of the people abusing me had ever set up any petition highlighting the plight of special needs children. In my mind if we offer the correct support in childhood adulthood can become easier for these individuals but here i was getting emailed loads of abuse for trying to make a difference. I stopped my petition and lost faith in ever making any difference.

I could not get my breath at the vile comments some of these so called human beings were spouting.  Anyway there came the idea of a series of ebooks on personal experiences that could help others.

As a nurse  mother daughter sister I like to help others it is in my nature thats just how I am.

Dean

Dean is my brother he is a prolific drug user. He is in and out of jail he is not reliable but he asked me when my lad was tiny if he was autistic due to so many people he had seen diagnosed in adulthood in prison with the condition. He had read book after book on Autism I guess when your in a cell for 23 hours a day you get time to read . He may be a royal pain in the arse but he saw what I couldn't. He stayed out of trouble long enough to attend my wedding and was able to warn me it may be difficult day for Olly he really helped that day with Olly and told me again that he thought my lad was on the spectrum. The wedding was really hard for Olly he cried all day looking back now I feel guilty for putting him through it.

getting at here is the people society least expects to have intelligence are often knowledgeable don;t ever dismiss advice from the lay person everyone has different stories and experiences don't assume . We can all learn from each other.

Selective mutism

Heightened anxiety has led to Olly literally being silent and refusing to speak for up to 3 days straight. December is always a difficult month he doesn't want to talk to anybody and doesn't want to leave the house. He cries a lot chews clothes generally is not his happy self

The quiet spells are difficult you kind of don't know what to do our child locked in there own little world refusing to interact it happens a few times  year and is extreme the only common link is that December and September are often triggers back to school and Christmas may be extremely anxiety provoking. If I knew all the answers Autism would not be the so called jigsaw disease with parents and carers like me and you having to piece thinks together just to get somewhere.

future plans.

My boy is currently in a mainstream school with some 1-1 support. I take each school day as it comes sometimes he is struggling that much that I cannot understand how he can remain in mainstream school.

Then there are the weeks that he gets an award for trying hard.

Plans of how best to educate him things being tweaked, meetings phone calls appointments. Research , trial and error.

I do not know where we will be in another academic years time. I know one thing I will keep negative people out of our life and I will continue fighting to raise awareness of the square pegs we as a society expect to fit into round holes.

I will keep persevering with getting a full nights sleep

USEFUL RESOURCES (uk)

Cerebra Website
The national Autistic Society
Young minds website
Family fund

Acknowledgments

To my 2 beautiful children you make mommy proud each day everything i do is for you don't ever change who you are for nobody.

My parents and husband always there no matter what.

To my brother underneath it all is a lovely person I hope one day your path in life changes.

for the children who don't get invited to parties, the adults labelled as quirky and odd. The people who can't tolerate changes to routine the little boys who will only wear seamless socks, the little girls who are non verbal but ca speak with their eyes you are all amazing you are just wired up differently.

Thank you for reading .

www.ingramcontent.com/pod-product-compliance
Lightning Source LLC
Chambersburg PA
CBHW061240180526
45170CB00003B/1378